After Covid-19...
What?

Peter Kirk

Dedication

To Dr Li Wenliang of Wuhan Central Hospital, Hubei Province, China, and all the medical staff around the world who have worked tirelessly to save lives during the Covid-19 pandemic.

May those who have died rest in peace.

Contents

Part One
Setting the Scene

Chapter 1
Posing the Questions

In 1974 the Spanish government garrotted two men convicted of terrorism. That the Spanish state could strangle criminals to death less than fifty years ago seems almost unbelievable. However, that was the Spain of General Francisco Franco, the Fascist leader who won the Spanish Civil War in the 1930s. In the mid-1970s Franco was coming to the end of his life and the question was frequently asked: "After Franco, what?" In the event, when he died Prince Juan Carlos was crowned king and, over the succeeding few years, steered the country through to democracy and later into the European Common Market: a success story.

In Eastern Europe another elderly dictator was coming to the end of his life. Marshal Tito had led the Yugoslavian resistance fighters against Hitler during the Second World War. When peace came, he established a less Moscow dependent version of Communism than the other east European states. The problem was that multi-ethnic Yugoslavia coalesced around his personality and political acumen. Again, the question was asked: "After Tito, what?" Following his death thousands died in civil wars, as Yugoslavia fell apart.

Two crises. Two very different results. Spain, despite its multi-ethnic tensions, held together, Yugoslavia did not. The world now faces a pandemic, the like of which we have not known in living memory, if ever. It has spread at lightning speed around the globe, mainly affecting the rich and middle-income countries of the world. As I write, we have still to see how Africa and South Asia will fare. Some commentators say the world will never be the same again.

With social distancing becoming the main weapon used to prevent the spread of the virus, economic life, locally and internationally, nearly ground to a halt. In less than six weeks the world economic system fell to pieces. Rich countries put undreamed of stimulus packages in place to prop up economic life and livelihoods. How these measures will be paid for is an unutterable question. Tourism disappeared and international travel, as well as travel within countries, has virtually ceased, except for transport of essential goods. Motorway traffic ceased. Airlines are going bust and the oil industry is running out of places to store surplus production. The world has never seen anything like it.

When Wall Street crashed in October 1929, it was only gradually over the succeeding months and years that the true enormity of the crisis emerged. As tariffs rose, trade declined and with depressed prices, stimulus to trade vanished. What is going to happen today? Can the virus be brought under control quickly enough for economies to re-open and will they bounce back as quickly as they have died? Has human society been so disturbed that until a vaccine is widely available, life cannot return to anything like normality? Do we want to return to the old normality or has the crisis shown that it was essentially broken anyway?

Yet there is a silver lining in all this. Air pollution is at record low levels. The sky is so clear that the people of Pakistan can see the Himalayas for the first time in decades. Delhi's smog has dissipated. During the Chinese lockdown people saw blue sky for the first time in years. The production of greenhouse gases has been decimated. Marshall Burke of Stamford University reckons that in China alone lower emissions have saved the lives of 1,400 children and 51,700 adults. The planet is breathing a sigh of relief. But have we already done too much damage for this to make any difference and will pollution levels be back to their fetid normal in a few weeks, or months at most?

As I write, the world's pause button has been pressed. Despite all the undoubted pain we are suffering, not least the tens of thousands of deaths which might have been avoided, we have an unprecedented opportunity to ask *where to from here*? Can we challenge economic orthodoxy and present a set of new possible narratives to the world? Is this the death of the neoliberal Washington Consensus or are those in political and economic power too strong to allow meaningful change? Whatever the answer to these and other questions, now is the time to think of alternatives, to debate possibilities, and to stimulate a multifaceted response in civil society. Let us create a groundswell of debate before the politicians and economic movers and shakers dictate our future according to their traditional short-term paradigms. Let us ask the question: "After Covid-19…What?"

Chapter 2
Covid-19 … Just what is it?

Very simply, it is a set of pathological conditions, generally centred around the lungs, caused by a newly discovered *Coronavirus*. There are seven very common forms of this type of pathogen circulating in human populations, some of which are usually associated with the common cold. *The World Health Organisation* (WHO) has called this one SARS-CoV-2 as it shares some features with the virus that causes Severe Acute Respiratory Syndrome (SARS) and Middle East Respiratory Syndrome (MERS). Though it seems more infectious, it causes less acute symptoms in most people. For some, elderly people and those with pre-existing conditions however, it can cause potentially fatal, lower respiratory tract infections. It is sometimes also associated with liver or kidney damage and acute heart disease as well as gastrointestinal symptoms like diarrhoea. Thus, unlike SARS and MERS, Covid-19 can present itself as multi-system breakdown in the body. It has also been seen to target the upper pulmonary lobe causing breathlessness (dyspnoea with hypoxia). Yet at the other end of the spectrum some people can be asymptomatic, appearing completely well, but can still be infectious. Around eighty percent of confirmed cases have only mild symptoms and the vast majority of people recover.

On January 10th China released genome sequencing data on SARS-CoV-2, which has become the basis for the race to create a vaccine. This was further confirmed by studies of oropharyngeal specimens taken from a Nepali student returning from Wuhan to Kathmandu and analysed in Hong Kong, which showed a 99.99% match.

This data and other studies of SARS-CoV-2 structure and behaviour have given us some clues as to why this virus is particularly easy to spread and can have such severe effects on the human body once it has infected a person. Like the original SARS virus, it is generally spherical with spike proteins on its outside. In the case of this new coronavirus these are particularly well adapted to latching onto our own ACE2 proteins. With the help of an enzyme called Furin, the spike proteins then split apart, and the infection builds up. Exactly how this happens is not yet clear, but it may be that as the virus replicates and kills more cells, these fall into the lower airways, carrying the virus with them. The resulting build-up of fluid in the lungs then restricts breathing.

This outline of the virus's behaviour seems to point to the need for early, extensive availability of testing in order to start symptomatic treatment as early as possible. This will limit the virus's ability to latch itself into the body's cells and move down to the lower pulmonary system, where it causes pneumonia, which is particularly difficult to treat.

What about Treatment and Vaccination?

Since the discovery and manufacture of penicillin and a raft of other antibiotics, respiratory conditions are generally considered to be treatable. Early-on, Chinese doctors found that Covid-19 did not respond to SARS treatment regimes, and the high death toll is partly due to the lack of any treatment to slow the onset of serious complications while the body's immune system fights the virus. On April 29th *The Lancet* reported that a virus inhibitor, Remdesivir, produced by the US company Gilead had some marginal effect in speeding recovery from Covid-19, but this Chinese study was inconclusive. Since then, trials in the Unites States have led to this drug being licenced for emergency use (*Guardian Weekly May 8th*). What this shows is that we are at the beginning of a drug development journey. Doctors are saying it is like the early days of HIV-

Aids. Remdesivir has some positive effects and drug companies will therefore consider it worth investing in research to find other treatments. *The Lancet* (May 8th) reported a study of a triple combination therapy using interferon beta-1b, lopinavir–ritonavir, and ribavirin, which shortened recovery times for mild to moderate cases of Covid-19. We can expect cocktails of antiviral drugs to be used in the future, much the same way as antiretrovirals are used to help Aids patients manage their conditions. However, there is no sign of a cure for Covid-19.

There has been much talk about the search for a vaccine. According to the BBC (23rd April) 80 different groups around the world are working towards this Holy Grail. As we have often been told, vaccine development usually takes many years of careful testing, including animal and human trials. In this case, solid trials are vital if there are to be mass vaccination campaigns. The assumption seems to be that nearly everyone needs to have it. It is usually said that at least 95% coverage is needed to see a disease eliminated.

There is no room for short cuts. With the power of today's social media, if there is one rumour of serious side-effects or its failure to work, all today's efforts could be to no avail. We are told that a vaccine will take between 12 and 18 months to produce and there is a huge question about who will pay for it. In the 2014-16 West African Ebola crisis, 11,325 people was the reported death toll. A vaccine had been under development for 10 years, but without an affluent market, pharmaceutical companies were unwilling to invest enough for the vaccine to be ready when Ebola erupted. A year into the crisis, when it was used, it was nearly 100% successful. Had it been available earlier, many lives could have been saved.

Maybe this time, when the rich countries are crying over their collapsing economies, there will be enough of a profit motive to fund these eighty groups of dedicated scientists long enough to enable them to complete their work. Yet an even more important question is, *who will pay for the poor south to be vaccinated?* If there is one thing that this crisis has taught us, it is that **we are one world**: a few disparate clusters of infections in Wuhan became a global pandemic in under two months, as the world scrambled to work out what was happening and what to do about it.

We shall return to the question of unpreparedness later. In the context of vaccination, we need to realise that there is not just a moral imperative for both poor and rich alike to be vaccinated, but a sustainable future demands it. The rich countries cannot imagine that life can return to normal behind a wall of vaccine. If large areas of the world are left unvaccinated, it is likely that SARS-CoV-2 will mutate again and again, rendering vaccines repeatedly useless. It is therefore imperative that for world survival we begin now to put the structures in place to enable enough vaccine to be produced and made available at point of need, not rationed according to market forces. Whether it is through the WHO or stakeholders such as the *Coalition for Epidemic Preparedness Innovations* (CEPI) there must be a coordinated international response, so that when clinical trials are complete, vaccines can be hastened into production and released world-wide. Hitherto, the USA has taken on a major part of the WHO funding burden, but now, as its government withdraws once more from its international responsibilities, other countries will need to step up to the plate. Unless this is done, the gains we have seen from lockdowns and the pain endured in thousands of households amidst collapsing economic life, will unravel as new strains of the virus advance across the globe and social life disintegrates.

All this may seem alarmist. Surely, you say, once we've beaten it through social distancing, and testing and tracing regimes, the job is done. Not so, without determined cooperation to build a global vaccination system and epidemiological response regime, even if this Coronavirus appears to be beaten, we will not be ready for the next sickness to challenge the world. "Let's hope we're ok" does not suffice for building a sustainable future.

Chapter 3
Covid-19.... How? When? Where?

In order to talk about the future, we need to be clear about the past. Our preparations for future epidemics need to be informed by our knowledge of this and past diseases.

A paper published in the *Lancet* and studies by the WHO show that Covid-19 was established in the human population of Wuhan, Hubei province, China by early December 2019. On 7th January the Chinese National Institute of Viral Disease Control and Prevention (IVDC) confirmed that they had isolated a *Novel Coronavirus* as the cause of mysterious viral respiratory conditions which had come to light in Hubei. Throughout December small numbers of patients with serious respiratory disease symptoms continued emerged. Some of them were mistakenly diagnosed as suffering from SARS, as no other diagnosis was available. On December 30th Dr Li Wenliang of the Wuhan Central Hospital communicated via *WeChat* with Alumni about a cluster of seven patients diagnosed with SARS who had not responded to treatment and had been quarantined. On January 3rd he was summoned to the Wuhan State Security Bureau and made to sign a confession to "making false comments by announcing the confirmation of 7 cases of SARS at the Huanan Seafood Wholesale Market" that had "severely disturbed the social order".

During December and the first days of January the picture was confused both within the medical and scientific community and the state apparatus. It was not until 20th January 2020 that human to human transmission was confirmed by the China National Health Commission, a cabinet level committee responsible for national health policies. President Xi Jinping announced "people's lives and health should be given top priority and the spread of the outbreak should be resolutely curbed."

The same day the USA and South Korea reported their first cases to the WHO. In the next few days evidence of human to human transfer in Singapore emerged. On January 22nd Hong Kong and Macau reported their first cases. January 27th saw the first confirmed case in Canada. The following day Thailand reported 14 cases. January 31st saw the first cases in the UK and Russia.

By the end of January China's Hubei province had effectively been quarantined and travel within China was severely curtailed. For China to take such measures, effectively preventing Spring Festival celebrations and family reunions, indicated the severity of the situation.

A month later the official WHO figures set global infections at 83,652 confirmed cases, which was probably an underestimate, but shows the speed of global transmission. Fifty-one countries had reported cases. On March 11th WHO chief Dr Tedros Adhanom Ghebreyesus said the number of cases outside China had increased 13-fold in two weeks, confirming that this was indeed a pandemic.

The virus had by then severely affected several countries way beyond China. On 19th March the number of Covid-19 deaths in Italy had risen above the registered Chinese death toll. By April 27th Italy had 197,675 cases and 26,644 deaths, though over 60 thousand had recovered. Spain was similarly badly hit, with large numbers of deaths in aged-care facilities. By 27th April there had been 226,629 cases and 23,190 deaths. By the same date the U.S.A. had registered 928,619 cases and 52,459 deaths. India had 27,890 registered cases and 881 deaths. At the time of writing, we wait to see what the future holds for India, Sub-Saharan Africa and other less developed areas of the world.

What this timeline demonstrates is that the superfast spread of the virus took the Chinese and the world by surprise. The similarity of the symptoms and the pathogen to

SARS created early confusion in the scientific and medical community, which was compounded by the propensity for officials in the Chinese security apparatus to try to control the flow of information. We will turn later to a consideration of future actions that will speed-up both detection and responses to future epidemics.

Where did SARS-CoV-2 come from and how did it invade the human world?

The most commonly circulated story is that the Covid-19 pathogen came from the Huanan Seafood Wholesale Market in Wuhan, because the first cluster of cases was associated with the market. A 57 year old worker from the market first showed symptoms on 10th December. There is therefore a strong suggestion that the virus originated in an animal from this "wet market", maybe a bat or an illegally traded creature such as a pangolin. This market was closed on 1st January and sanitised, so any definite connection is now impossible to prove. What we do know is that large numbers of similar viruses circulate amongst wild animals and are capable of mutating and jumping into humans. Dr Stephen Turner from Melbourne's Monash University considers that bats could have acted as an intermediary, but the connection with the Huanan Market is only circumstantial. An article in the *Journal of Medical Virology* also casts doubt on the pangolin connection.

Interestingly, one of the earliest laboratory-confirmed cases, was an elderly Alzheimer's sufferer who rarely went out and had no connection with the market. So, it may be that the virus had jumped to humans some time previously and the present pandemic had several origins. The pathogen just needed to create a large enough pool of infection to enable large scale transmission to begin.

Another source of SARS-CoV-2 has also been suggested and has been championed by the White House. The latter has claimed there is strong evidence to connect the virus with a Wuhan laboratory and that it is the result of genetic manipulation. Conspiracy theorists go further and claim that the Chinese government deliberately allowed it to escape in order to poison the world. Despite the seriousness of these claims, no concrete evidence has been presented to the public.

In response, scientists and biosecurity experts have examined the evidence. Looking at virus mutations which allowed it to jump the species barrier, they conclude that the evidence points strongly to natural random changes rather than laboratory based genetic manipulation. Studies of the SARS-CoV-2 g-nome also suggest gradual accretion of anatomical changes due to environmental interaction. There are none of the tell-tale signs of reverse genetic engineering typically left behind by laboratory tampering. (Los Angeles Times, May 9th). Evidence described in the journal *Nature*

Medicine and the *Journal of Virology* fundamentally undercut the conspiracy theories.

Virus mutations are common, which is why influenza vaccines need to be constantly updated to take account of the changes in the g-nome. The SARS-CoV-2 pathogen is relatively stable, which is good news for vaccine development. However, studies (Science Alert, May 6th) at Arizona State University and Los Alamos National Laboratory, (Science Alert, May 6th), show minor mutations which may help to make the virus more transmissible than the original Wuhan virus. Despite this unwelcome news, studies show only very minor changes and many of these do not aid the development of the virus.

Chapter 4
What Happened to the World
Economy and Why?

The collapse of economic life has been horrifyingly sudden, but why? Let's now look at how our modern world operates.

The International Monetary Fund's *World Economic Outlook* published in January of this year stated "Global growth is projected to rise from an estimated 2.9 percent in 2019 to 3.3 percent in 2020 and 3.4 percent for 2021…[and]…market sentiment has been boosted by tentative signs that manufacturing activity and global trade are bottoming out." Not a rosy picture, but it was business as usual. Geopolitical challenges received cautious mention, but choppy waters could be navigated.

Within two months the world economy had collapsed like a house of cards. Amidst the language of "monetary policy,… advanced economies…[and]…emerging markets" there had been no mention that people's health might just possibly be important. Suddenly the card labelled *healthy populations* slipped from its place and everything else came tumbling down. China's great manufacturing behemoth ground to a halt in the face of lockdown. Tourism disappeared from world economies and aeroplanes ceased to fly, while cruise ships became Covid-19 breeding grounds. India's government told everyone to stay at home, but forgot about the millions in the informal workforce whose homes were either on the streets or several hundred kilometres away, and…oh dear! They couldn't go back to their villages because the trains had been told to stop moving!

The Maori people of New Zealand have a traditional saying, *He aha te mea nui o te ao. He tāngata, He tāngata. He tāngata* . **What is the most important thing in the world? It is people. It is people. It is people.** Surely this is another lesson we have learned from this crisis. Economies run on people: even when they have been shunted off to work from home, it is still people who make it all work. Where, over the last weeks, has all that talk of automation been? However much people are undervalued, underpaid, and overworked, when they are suddenly unable to work, because public health demands social distancing, we realise that people are the key engine of the whole economy. Without people, it stops. What is more, the economy exists not for the sake of the invisible hand of the market, but for people.

The founding fathers of the United States of America began their constitution by describing the inalienable rights of people, not property. The world economic system, based as it is on the ownership of capital and the rule of law, is only as strong as its ability to preserve the lives and welfare of citizens. When capitalism fails to protect the people, it is in danger of precipitating its own destruction. Given the world economic collapse we have witnessed, it is arguable that our economic system has failed to enable governments to fulfil their first responsibility: to protect their people.

Before we ask what economic changes need to be made in the post Covid-19 world, let us first explore why this collapse happened at all. Did the world economy have to collapse in the way it has done? Is it weakly structured and could it be reformed?

For as long as there has been trade, different areas and nations have learned to specialise in the production and sale of specific commodities. Such specialisation produces income, which in turn is used to stimulate more production and through this *multiplier effect* economies grow. This creates confidence in a cycle of growth, which in turn creates more wealth and generates capital to invest in further wealth creation. This specialisation works according to what is often called the *law of comparative advantage.* In the modern world the advantage belongs to the most efficient and cheapest global producers.

Whereas this system is good up to a point, there comes a stage when it creates supply chains which originate in very few countries. In 2012, figures from the *International Observatory on Economic Complexity* show that seven far Eastern countries produced 96% of the global supply of integrated circuits. In 2018 *World Footwear* reported that nine out of every ten pairs of shoes were made in Asia. Of course, it is well known that face mask production centres on China and east Asia. Ventilator production is concentrated in the USA, China, Sweden, Switzerland, and Germany covering between 70% and 90% of production in 2019. Britain had one small company making ventilators. World Trade Organisation (WTO) and the European Union rules have made it difficult for countries to protect small, local manufacturers who are unable to compete with larger international producers. Efficiency has continuously been construed to mean the same as low cost and national governments have been refused permission to provide financial or other support to local producers. A wider understanding of efficiency would include the strategic need to protect essential industries, especially in the medical sector. Short-term efficiency may mean buying from the manufacturer offering the cheapest product. Long-term efficiency means having local alternative supplies of products available in case the cheaper product is not available, so that efficiencies gained in the short-term can be sustained.

For too long, the world economy has been run on the hope that annual GDP growth will continue to keep up with population growth, perpetually looking at shorter- and shorter-term indicators such as quarterly forecasts of economic performance. In 2008 the world economy fell over because of the race for short-term gains from sub-prime mortgages and associated financial investment tools that few people understood. We obviously have not learned some fundamental lessons.

The first of these is that our supply chains of essential products must not rely on availability from only a few countries. As western countries have increasingly moved manufacturing off-shore, Europe and America have lost strategic skills. Britain's ability to make respirators is so diminished that a consortium of engineering firms has been brought together to design and produce them from scratch. For a long time, it has been believed that manufacturing can be off-loaded and replaced with service industries and the world of data gathering and control. This crisis has revealed a truth that the virtual world of digital technology is something of a chimera. The world of the virtual reality headset is great fun and has valuable applications for both physical and mental health, but it will not save you when you cannot breathe. Governments must ensure that manufacturing expertise and plant are maintained in enough regions around the world to maintain supplies of vital health equipment at times of crisis.

The second and even more fundamental lesson involves a change of mind-set. As individuals, we live from our heads and our hearts. What we think and feel govern our lives. So it is for society as a whole. No-one would say that governments have no role to play when it comes to defence against military aggression; nobody would seriously out-source a nation's defence. Yes, private companies manufacture weapons and sometimes mercenaries serve alongside our national armies, but no government can seriously entrust defence to market forces. Yet in other areas of strategic national capacity, that is what has happened. As we have seen, the supply of respirators is a case in point. In 2006, under President Bush, the U.S. administration was warned of the shortfall in ventilators and a $6 million dollar contract was awarded to *Newport Medical Instruments*, a small Californian company. Due to a buy-out by a larger competitor, the ventilators were never made. The market failed to provide what was required. Even worse, in the United States today, as doctors and nurses work hard to save lives, medical workers are being laid off, because the usual stream of money-making operations has dried up, as hospitals are inundated with Covid-19 patients. The market driven United States healthcare system has failed to deliver the goods. There is effectively no public healthcare system based on the needs of patients. The whole system is structured around profits.

So, just as governments make strategic decisions about national defence needs, post Covid-19, we must look across the range of national and international needs and ensure that there is a balance of priorities in decision making so that the preservation of people's lives and wellbeing takes front and centre stage in strategic planning.

We have had a wake-up call. This is the end of the totally *laiser-faire* economy. It is not a call to abandon capitalism and swing to socialism and an all-out planned economy, but it is a call for governments to be active in planning how their economies can meet the essential needs of the people. It is not bleeding-heart socialism, but hard-headed economics. It is already feared that we are headed for a depression worse than in the 1930s, so we must plan against future economic collapse. Every country needs to look at weak points primarily in the supply chains for food and medical technology, pharmaceuticals and other products essential to national survival and wellbeing.

We all know that the need for social distancing is the immediate cause of factories, food outlets and shops having to close. Yet these extreme measures have been taken because the strategic, health related manufacturing industries and stockpiles of necessary technology and equipment were not there to meet the demands of a crisis that experts had said was bound to come. We were not prepared. Had resources and systems been in place to address the appearance of the first Covid-19 case, such a severe economic shutdown could have been avoided.

We may not be going to war, but there needs to be strategic preparedness for the future. The challenges presented by SARS, MERS, Avian Flu, H1N1 and Ebola are not going to end when Covid-19 is brought under control. As I write, people are already talking about another spike in infections as lockdowns are eased. I will turn later to the international response needed to address the likelihood of potential future pandemics and the future shape of economic life. Here, I just want to reiterate that if we are going to protect ourselves from future economic collapse due to another pandemic or a food crisis, we need an economic strategy which will enable us to plan our future and not just leave it to the free market.

Part Two
Shaping the Future

Chapter 5
What about public health?

Despite China's well publicised failings in the early weeks of the epidemic, it needs to be recognised that once through the initial confusion, China acted with great speed and efficiency to stem the spread of the virus and treat its own citizens. This is not to ignore the many heart-rending stories of people searching for treatment for sick relatives. Eventually the authorities should answer for these failures.

However, once lockdown in Wuhan was achieved, infection rates slowed quickly and initial numbers of infections beyond China's borders were few. Countries and territories which acted quickly to contain domestic spread of the disease through testing and contact tracing, namely South Korea, Taiwan, Singapore, Iceland, Germany and Hong Kong were successful in reducing local disease and death rates. As we look to the future, we need to study in detail how these countries operated and why they were successful. Focussing on examples of good practice will be much more fruitful in building successful future action, than pointing fingers and entering into blame games. Let us not forget that within 3 days of isolating the SARS-CoV-2 g-nome, Chinese scientists had shared it with the world. This information is the basis of our search for effective vaccines. The time for enquiries into what went wrong will come, but let us allow space for international co-operation while we are still struggling to deal with the pandemic.

Moving forward, let us return to the challenge of providing for future health needs. As people have died of Covid-19, others have succumbed to strokes, cancer, heart disease and a myriad of other conditions. Some health planners are already talking about developing parallel health systems, one focussed on public health crises, structured around epidemiology, and the other meeting on-going general and specialised health requirements. Such an approach would mean that we are ready, nationally and internationally, with the tools and expertise to meet the challenges of future pandemics without an accompanying societal collapse.

One important tool is research into the link between immunity and nutrition. The truism "we are what we eat" may be simplistic, but one key piece of evidence from statistics about deaths during the pandemic is that people with brown skins seem more likely to die than their Caucasian neighbours. In Louisiana, it was claimed that this was related to poverty and lifestyle choices. However, evidence of a high proportion of deaths amongst medical staff from ethnic minorities in the U.K. and the U.S.A. points in a more complex and potentially more helpful direction. A link has been shown between low vitamin D-levels in people with dark skins and increased Covid-19 morbidity. Particularly in cooler climates, dark skinned people do not absorb vitamin-D from sunlight as well as their light skinned compatriots. The United States National Centre for Biotechnology Information (NCBI) identifies Vitamin-D as a key factor in the operation of our immune systems. Testing for vitamin-D and ensuring that people have vitamin rich diets will help people to fight future pandemics.

Importantly, national public health systems need to be linked globally, so that barriers to information sharing and co-operation are cut to a minimum. Already at the professional level relationships exist through international journals and specialised professional bodies. It is at the governmental level that change is needed. One way of doing this would be the signing of an international public health treaty, putting public health into the hands of a supranational body, with powers to enforce its decisions. This has been done before in different contexts. When the world realised the damage Chlorofluorocarbons were doing in the atmosphere, the Montreal Protocol was signed in 1987 to stop their manufacture and use. Further back, in 1959, the international Antarctic Treaty was signed by all countries with interests in Antarctica, in order to prevent geopolitical competition and industrial exploitation in the area.

Given the ego-dominated state of international politics at present, a return to such meaningful international co-operation seems doubtful. It would, however, be hoped that the collapse of the world's economies caused by Covid-19 might breed a sense of cooperation even for the sake of national self-interests. Establishment of such a global public health body would be one pillar of a new and stronger set of world social, economic and political institutions.

Such a world body, whether an extension of the WHO or a new entity, would need to develop clear, shared protocols on pandemic management. It seems clear that aggressive testing and contact tracing are keys to early management of disease outbreaks. Yet few countries made this a priority. Britain's early approach of treating the infection in a similar way to annual waves of influenza was soon shown to be a desperately serious mistake. Clear, internationally agreed public health guidelines are needed in order to facilitate swift and effective action in the likely event of future public health emergencies. Failures in the WHO's effectiveness were structural rather than personal. It needs continuously to perform diplomatic balancing acts to keep on side with countries, because it does not have the power to implement a robust response to the health emergencies it identifies around the world. An international organisation resourced and empowered to monitor epidemiological risks, and act rapidly to isolate dangerous pathogens as they emerge, is vital to the world's future health and economic and social welfare.

What about the next pandemic?

You might shriek in horror and say, "We haven't even finished with this one yet, why should we be planning for the next?" But that is the point of this book. While our minds are concentrated on this present horror, we have the impetus to prepare for the future. If we do not think now, it is all too easy to let those who hold the levers of power to go back to their economic short-termism, coupled with the *hope it doesn't happen* syndrome. What in the antipodes is called the *she'll be right!* attitude.

This is the time for *joined up thinking*. Preparing for the future is not just about having the structures in place to defend ourselves when the enemy attacks. Efforts to find dangerous new pathogens need to be organised and resourced so we can hollow out the enemy before it reaches us. Coronaviruses are Zoonotic pathogens which jump the species barrier between animals and humans. In the last 30 years at least 50 viruses have done this. In 2009 the USAID *Predict Project* was established to identify sources of future epidemics, isolating 1,200 animal viruses including 160 coronaviruses. The natural world contains millions and millions of viruses which pose a threat to humans. Bats, in particular, have been identified as sources, most likely because they often live in close proximity to humans. It is thought that Ebola resulted from a boy being bitten by a bat.

In less developed countries people often live close to animals and as natural habitat is increasingly lost, animals and humans are competing more and more for territory. Hence the risk of viruses jumping to humans is growing. Those working in the field of rural epidemiology around the world believe it is vital to have people working on the ground with local populations to identify dangers and engage in health education, thereby helping people to live safely alongside wildlife. Such fieldworkers are our first line of defence against viral transmission. A boy in a rural village can be infected by a bite from a bat. He then travels to a town, and while selling goods in a market, infects a businessman. The businessman goes to the capital city and stays in a hotel, infecting others, one of whom flies to New York carrying an unknown pathogen and an epidemic/pandemic may have begun. Mercifully, wide-scale disease transmission usually requires the development of a local cluster of cases, which alerts local authorities to impending danger before international transmission occurs.

The last twenty years have seen key universities around the world looking into the dangers of pathogens developing in animals and transferring to humans. This danger is increased by the international trade in endangered species, as this is by nature hidden from the authorities and therefore not regulated by health and hygiene standards. This current crisis raises important public health questions as to how research into the sources of future pandemics amongst wildlife populations may be resourced and organised. The way in which wild animals have so quickly come back into what seemed to be *our* space during lockdown shows that we really do share this world with a host of not too distant neighbours. We need to find safe ways of thriving together.

Zoonotic infections will certainly continue to proliferate and with globalisation, the danger of further pandemics remains. We therefore have a clear choice, either to abandon a globalised economy, with its potential for wealth creation, or to incorporate widespread virus identification into our future strategic planning.

Unfortunately, the Trump administration discontinued the *Predict Project* in 2019, which had scientists working in Wuhan laboratories, as well as in 30 other countries about three months before the emergence SARS-CoV-2. Smaller projects run by universities around the world need to be expanded and linked in a globally coordinated approach. Viruses must be identified, and their g-nomes isolated, so that when zoonotic infections occur public health authorities can identify and isolate those infected. Community based health education and epidemiological research into social and economic practices which encourage transmission, will also help to reduce infections.

If this approach to strategic epidemiology is followed, pathogens and infections will be identified long before extreme measures of social distancing and economic shut down are necessary because infections will be firewalled before community transfer can take place. Putting this work in the hands of a strong international body, created by international treaty and beyond the reach of politicians, would help to ensure that this defensive system of pathogenic detection and control is created and maintained.

Chapter 6
Will we meet again?

In her address to Britain and the Commonwealth, Queen Elizabeth II evoked the wartime spirit and assured us that we would meet again. Social isolation cannot be humanity's future, nor is it possible in many parts of the world: the slums of Kolkata and Nairobi do not allow it, nor is it desirable. People need to meet together. We need to hug our neighbours sometimes. As I write this, some of us are beginning to come out of lockdown, while others are prolonging its pain in search of the public health benefits. On the other hand, some high-profile figures have refused to believe it has any benefits and believe that the pain is too much to bear.

What will social interaction look like and what should it look like? Have we said goodbye to the handshake, or will it be reserved for greetings between friends and family who know they are free from infections? What about kisses on cheeks? Of course, those who greet with a bow or hands together and a nod of the head have less to worry about. Will we see the adoption of such greetings more widely across the world?

These are arguably less important issues than the question of how, where and for what purposes we can gather together again. Are we just going to see sports matches played behind closed doors and live streamed on pay-as-you-watch media? What about the arts: concerts, drama, dance and the visual arts? Maybe we can visit galleries as long as we remain two metres apart!

No doubt the return to something like normality will be gradual. We will slowly loosen up. Greetings will be negotiated, tentatively at first. It will all depend on local conditions. If the virus seems to have been kicked into touch, then we might relax. Yet, while a vaccine and effective treatments remain some way off, we will be on our guard. I expect it will take a long time before physical distancing is abandoned in the shops and I doubt if the Perspex screens will ever go away.

So much of life is social, or at least it was. We started with kindergarten and then school and maybe university. We went to work on building sites, and in office, shops, factories etc. Social media may have changed life to some degree, but was still a supplement to physical interaction, rather than a wholesale replacement for it. Has Covid-19 changed our interactive world? Has it speeded up the move towards life structured around digital devices? Zoom has profited hugely as people have been unable to meet together physically. Will much of our physical interaction for education, worship and work be replaced by Zoom meetings and other forms of video conferencing? Why leave our warm houses, take a bus, sit in a traffic jam, or walk through the rain, when we can meet online? Will our classes or churches meet predominantly online and only occasionally in physical spaces? And if this happens, will we need so many private physical buildings or will we learn to share communal spaces? Who knows? These are open questions and different contexts will have different answers, but there is room for a lot of creativity.

Yet, is it enough just to accept what comes along? Should we not be more proactive in demanding health measures and the development of technology that facilitates getting back to physical proximity and interaction. As fast, easy to use, testing technologies are developed we need to make sure that high streets and shopping malls have testing facilities available to all.

Yet this is also a double-edged sword. Along with testing goes the need to trace the contacts of those whose tests are positive. Test, trace, isolate is the maxim, and along with this goes increased surveillance. In the context of keeping us all safe, who would argue with this? But there is a strange feature of human nature. Once people are given power to influence the lives of others, this leads to an enhanced desire for control of their lives. Surveillance helps in the exercise of political control.

During the present crisis, apps have been developed for mobile phones which monitor people's movements in order to map contact with people who may be carrying the virus. Google and Apple have worked together to produce such an app. Others have also joined the field. What is uncertain is whether these systems will work. How many people need to be using them for them to be effective? How much data do they store? Where does it go to and for how long is it kept? The Google/Apple system is decentralised and does not share names and addresses. Some other systems do, and in some places that information is shared with the police, and use of the system is compulsory. It is easy to see that these systems could easily be used for purposes much less legitimate than public health protection. We will meet again, but who will be watching?

Finally, what about work? Many work situations demand physically shared space. A factory assembly line cannot be operated remotely from home, unless it is entirely robotic and even then, there will always be some human involvement. Shops require assistants. Banks may seem like they want to retire all their tellers, but queues for personal assistance remain. Building sites require builders.

Yet during the Covid-19 crisis many people have started to work from home and are very happy doing so. Managers have often worried that working from home would lead to inefficiency: workers would be out of their reach and idle away their time watching Netflix! However, reports so far suggest that the results have been good for business. Have we been jolted into a new office culture? Is the online, video conference office going to become the predominant social situation for the "white collar" workforce. CEO of Twitter, Jack Dorsey, has already said employees can work from home 'forever'. Maybe staff will never meet again around the photocopier for a coffee?

Yet, is it enough just to accept what comes along? Should we not be more proactive in demanding health measures and the development of technology that facilitates getting back to physical proximity and interaction. I believe that there are serious reasons for social distancing not becoming the norm: it is dangerous for society. As we are physically distanced from each other, it is easier to put social and personal needs at a distance. The stay home, locked down elderly lose their voice just like those who are stashed away in aged-care facilities. It is only when you sit down with a homeless person on the pavement that you go beyond the concept to the person, and find a rich life of valuable experience waiting to be shared. We will all be poorer if we cannot socialise. It is therefore important to work hard towards the resumption of sharing physical space. We may need to pressure politicians to make resources available to facilitate this process. Undoubtedly part of this is the development of easy to use, virus testing kits and the infrastructure for their use. There needs to be a mind-set that it is good to meet, that we need to meet and that we will make it happen safely, even before vaccinations become available. At the same time, let's watch out that we protect our privacy.

Chapter 7
What could the post Covid-19 economy look like?

As I write this, the world economy is wrecked. A situation similar to the Great Depression is forecast. It is estimated that at least 36% of people are out of work globally. Millions upon millions of workers in the informal economies of the two thirds world (the poor south) have lost their precarious sources of income in a flash. Living hand to mouth means that if you don't work today, you don't eat tomorrow. The future looks dire. Even in the rich countries, millions of people live on the next paycheque. Even for those who have savings, any investment earnings are likely to be very low. The Bank of England's base rate was 0.1% when I last looked.

The most visible indicator of a world economic vacuum is the sudden departure of air traffic from our skies. According to *cntraveler.com,* by the end of April, there was a 95% reduction in usual passenger air traffic in the United States. In the Middle East, only 50 planes are flying at any one time, compared to a usual figure of 300. Emirates and Etihad have grounded nearly all their planes. IATA estimated a loss of $113bn in worldwide revenue. Cost cutting measures, including large scale redundancies, are in progress and bankruptcies are likely.

Due to lockdowns and border closures, tourism has virtually disappeared. The impact is felt most keenly within the travel and hospitality industries and the burden is falling hardest on poorer countries.

China has been the first country to get back to work. Yet on 17th April the BBC reported a 6.8% contraction in the Chinese economy, while consumer sales slid 15.8% in March (Bloomberg). On April 29th 77.3% of businesses had higher than 80% of their usual capacity utilisation rates (CNBC). It is early days, but global demand will have to pick up for China's economy to recover.

The post Covid-19 world economy depends on the ability of people world-wide to return to work. China has begun that process, while at the same time continuing social distancing, both at work and on public transport. For the world economy, these are the two key issues: how to return to work, while keeping everyone safe. If we cannot work safely, returning to work will lead to a further cycle of infection and consequent economic dislocation.

The ideal solution to this problem is of course the discovery of suitable vaccines so that we can interact physically without fear. Vaccines, however, are still likely to take at least a year to become available and world-wide immunisation will take some time. In the meantime, stringent health checks on workers entering premises and the maintenance of as much social distance as possible are undoubtedly the way forward. Easily used Covid-19 test kits giving results within minutes must obviously become ubiquitous around the world, especially in workplaces. Such tests are under development. This must also be linked with contact tracing, which will necessarily involve temporary infringement of privacy. The South Korean experience has shown us the value of such a regime. If it can help get us back to work, it is worth it. It is part of the paradigm shift to strategic thinking that will be vital to re-building life in the post Covid-19 world.

Working from home has been discussed above. It will be surprising if this crisis does not lead to its wide-scale embrace, though evidence from China shows that people used to traditional work practices in large organisations with hierarchical structures struggle with it. One result of this change is likely to be a lessening in demand for office accommodation, a lowering of business rents and a concomitant downturn in the private building industry.

What about Macro-economic Policy?

Economic health has always been built on confidence, especially since the demise of the *Gold Standard* as the foundation of the world's currencies. If companies believe that investment will result in profit, they will make investments. Confidence has vanished over-night. Who would invest in a new factory today, other than for ventilator, face mask, PPE equipment and vaccine production? At times of economic crisis there are three ways to artificially create confidence.

1. Encourage private investment
2. Monetary policy: increase the money supply by making borrowing cheaper
3. Increase net public spending

Private investment, as already noted, is usually dependent on consumer confidence which at the present time is severely depressed. It requires governmental action to stimulate it. Monetary policy is a non-starter. Interest rates can hardly go any lower. The danger is that they may soon be in negative territory. The United States Federal Reserve

Rate stood at 0.25% on 29th April. Cheap money is available to prop up struggling businesses, but who wants to invest?

We are therefore left with public spending. The approach is simple. When private sector money is draining from the system and recession or depression is on the horizon, governments pump money into their economies to create demand. The question is, how can this be done at this stage in history? Rich countries have already created sizeable stimulus packages to prop up businesses. New Zealand has sold Kiwi bonds to fund investment of NZ$12bn. On 25th March the U.S. Congress agreed a package of $2 trillion in Washington and more is on the way. European Union leaders have agreed a total of $540bn and Australia has pumped AU$213.6bn directly into social security and job and wage protection (Guardian March 31st). But all this is short-term cash. The hope is that it will ease things long enough for economies to re-open for business. People are hoping for a fast V-shaped recovery, which is looking less and less likely.

What about long-term economic revitalization? In the Great Depression of the 1930s the USA began to recover as a result of the New Deal. Public spending on large scale public works began to pull the country together, but by the late 1930s activity was slowing and they were looking at a double dip depression. It was the Second World War that launched the United States of America on its trajectory to become the world's economic superpower. Strategic economic wartime planning dragged America out of its hole.

Such strategic long-term spending is required now. The first obvious area of investment is in health infrastructure, technology and on-going supplies. Given its importance for the future physical and economic health of nations, this is an area in which private companies should have confidence in making investments. As outlined above, there needs also to be strategic examination of national life and priorities in order to identify areas where governmental investment support will help to guarantee supply of essential products at times of crisis.

This pause in economic life also gives us an opportunity to think about how we can stimulate the creation and development of new industries, and the further development of existing industries away from existing economic centres of power. For too long, economic power has been concentrated in a few hands. At the same time older industrial centres have been ignored. The resulting sense of frustration and disempowerment has caused the growth of illiberal populism. Let us take this opportunity to stimulate regional industrial regeneration.

As we look to the future there is need to harness the dynamic power of creativity. The figure of Captain, now Colonel, Tom determinedly plodding his way around the outside of his home to raise £32 million for the British National Health Service should be a defining image we take with us into the future. Independent creative spirits working together in civil society offer us a real way forward into our post Covid-19 future. However, people need to come together to help each other develop new and creative endeavours. Both governments and private capital have roles to play to fund small and medium scale income and employment generating projects birthed in the hearts of individuals and communities. This is therefore a time for a paradigm shift in thinking, into an era when creative entrepreneurial thinking is not the exception, but the expectation. As economies are rebuilt locally, nationally and internationally, we should not see this just happening for us through government initiatives, but resulting from a combined effort of people and communities, private industry and government spending.

Above and beyond these initiatives, governments need to look nationally and internationally at infrastructure. A large scale, long-term public spending programme is vital to the re-building of the international economy. Moreover, planning and commitment to it need to begin now, before so much more confidence is lost, and more businesses go to the wall.

This is where macro-planning interfaces with the micro-level. Business does not just need a lifeline now, but a road-map to recovery. Each business needs to develop a tailored regular virus-testing regime, with the ability to upload data to a national database, so that workers can get back to work. Finance needs to be made available to businesses as they re-build production, services and markets.

This is not a job for 6 months or a year down the road. Government securities from all around the world need to be pooled in order to back the sale of 10-year Covid-19 bonds as the basis for a global recovery fund. Working together we can finance world recovery. Individually we could fail. International cooperation will generate confidence for private capital to join the party.

We know that private capital is plenteous. Individuals and corporations have more available equity than the GDPs of some countries. In 2019 *Forbes* listed 2,153 billionaires with net wealth of $8.7trillion. These people are capable of underwriting the recovery of hundreds of thousands of small businesses. For this to happen we need two things. One is the creation of an atmosphere of expectation that the wealthy should at this time make their riches available for the benefit of all. This is not an expectation that they should just give their wealth away, but that they should use it to finance small and medium-sized business recovery. For many of these wealthy people, small business and fledgling enterprise is where they began, and they can now use their wealth and expertise to the benefit of all. Secondly, systems of support at local levels need to be created so that private capital, public finance and local small and medium sized businesses can be brought together to build the future.

As we re-build a people-centred economic model, there is a particular place for cooperative businesses. The strength of cooperatives is that their owners are usually involved in the day to day running of their businesses and their stake in success is directly linked to their own livelihoods. At this time, when seeing people back in long-term work takes priority over making short-term profits, the cooperative business model has the potential to be more community driven and ignite local creative power, because it can create ownership in the community. If we can build local economies with community roots, we can have more vibrant local economic life.

As we consider the shape of the future economy, let us not forget that economic collapse is usually the result of demand being taken out of the system. It is often triggered by one event such as the Wall Street Crash, the 2008 banking crisis, or a pandemic. One way to lessen the effects of such crises is for everyone to receive a *universal wage*. So, instead of having a benefit system for people in financial need, everyone receives a basic allowance, which enables them to pay for accommodation and cover other basic needs. As most people would be unhappy merely living on the basics, they would still want to work, but at times of crisis, individuals, families and the economy as a whole would be cushioned from extreme collapse.

In 2017-18 Finland rolled out a trial scheme which gave €560.00 a month to randomly selected citizens. There was a general increase in wellbeing and confidence amongst the participants and they did not abandon work and in some cases it helped them to accept lower paying jobs that they had previously rejected. So, at this time of crisis, I suggest that provision of a *universal wage* should be looked at again as a means to long-term economic prosperity.

In conclusion, the new economies require the following:

1. A structured public health environment based around regular virus-testing and national contact tracing strategies.

2. The urgent establishment of an international financial environment aimed at re-building business confidence through a system of ten-year bonds.

3. Government spending on a public health system designed to combat Covid-19 and other epidemics

4. Government support of strategic industries and infrastructure.

5. A creative partnership between public and private capital in support of small to medium sized enterprises.

6. Focus on rural and regional populations beyond the centres of political and economic power.

Chapter 8
What about Sport, Leisure and the Arts?

The second century Roman poet, Juvenal, bemoaned the populace's loss of civic virtue: "all they want is bread and circuses." The *circuses* he referred to, were the sports that took place in the Coliseum. Juvenal may not have had much time for sports, but there is no doubt that sports are integral to human societies everywhere. Every society has developed sports and now local and international sport is a key aspect of cultural life. Yet, suddenly sports have either disappeared or been reduced to the virtual arena.

Sport is not only an indispensable part of human life and society; it is big business. Powerful economic interests therefore will not let professional sport die, nor should they, but it is under threat. Sport depends on the crowds of spectators to generate income. While social distancing rules apply, how can basketball, football and cricket stadiums open again? How can people stand next to each other in crowds if one single person might be infected with Covid-19?

Social discipline and virus testing technology are the way forward. With enough investment, tests could be developed to give results within minutes. Once these tests are available spectators could attend testing centres set up in stadium car parks, remaining separate until they are cleared to enter the stadium. All this could be done electronically. Within a few months this technology could be available. If sports authorities want to speed the return to mass sporting activities, they could help to fund the development of these tests and the digital technology to facilitate their use in sporting and other facilities. The cost of tests could be factored into the cost of tickets. When mass tests such as these are available, they will no doubt cost much less than testing costs now. Creative thinking and 21st century technology could bring sports matches back more quickly than we think.

Already Bosch has developed a test which gives results in two and a half hours. We can expect this to be reduced. The BioMedomics COVID-19 IgM/IgG Rapid test is already available, gives results in 15 minutes and requires no specialised training for staff. However, this test may be unreliable because it depends on the detection of antibodies, which are only made a week to twelve days after infection. Therefore, some infected patients may not be identified. Other rapid testing systems are being developed around the world, including in New Zealand. The CRISP SARS-CoV-2 testing kit, developed by the University of California San Francisco and Mammoth Biosciences, uses gene targeting technology to identify the genetic signature of the SARS-CoV-2 g-nome, also contrasting it with a related coronavirus signature in order to guard against false results. The speed of these developments shows the valuable part testing can play in getting back to normal socialising even before a vaccine is available. Sporting organisations, governments and the medical technology industry need to establish strong working relationships in order to facilitate these developments. This is the kind of *joined-up thinking* that we need.

The situation is similar for the arts. Actors, musicians and dancers around the globe have had their livelihoods destroyed. Arts venues have closed their doors in response to social distancing restrictions. Some people have asked whether we will ever see a choir or symphony orchestra grace a stage again. How can crowds pack out the concerts of Elton John, Foo Fighters or Taylor Swift? Is crowd surfing a thing of the past and is the festival scene dead and gone?

We have to hope not. But more than that, we have to make sure that the arts will rise again. This is not just for the sake of practitioners. Art inspires us and helps us express our inner selves, reaching deep inside and helping us to discern who we are. Already, we have found singers, musicians and actors taking to the internet in order to encourage people during lockdown. Italians have been famously singing to each other from their balconies. The arts are a tool for the re-birth of communities after Covid-19.

Historically, artistic cultural expression did not begin amongst the bright lights of exotic venues, but in the stories and songs families and communities shared with each other. Can we not utilise the latent artistic hunger in all humanity to pull people together and stimulate creative expression? Is this not a period of world history which needs to be captured in story, song, drama and dance? There are opportunities for civil society to tell its story and reclaim the arts as part of the popular imagination.

Of course, there are also the professional artistic communities which inspire us by their creativity and expertise. They engender the *wow factor*, which the amateur sometimes struggles to create. However, maybe we have at this juncture an opportunity to bring the amateur and the professional together to speak into each other's lives and contexts. While major performing contracts are on hold, might professional musicians, actors and dancers not offer to perform in local communities, to smaller groups of people meeting within social distancing rules. Such communities might rarely see live performances and would have their spirits inspired, while the musicians would receive some financial return. There also needs to be creative use of digital media platforms such as Zoom. International and domestic conferences have reorganised themselves into webinars. Could the artistic world not do the same, offering a pay-to-view concert opportunity, plus a chance to join with performers in a webinar format? There could be the beginning of a new form of artistic engagement with the public. While Covid-19 has savagely disrupted artistic life, are not artists just the people to create new opportunities out of the ashes of the old.

Chapter 9
What of the Elephant in the Room?

Yes, there is an elephant in the room, and it is looking at us very suspiciously at present. I think the elephant fears it is going to be left out of this discussion altogether, as if Covid-19 has displaced it. If you listen to most of the news media, that is exactly what appears to have happened. You have guessed it: the natural environment.

The massive fall in emissions of greenhouse gases and the return of cleaner air is fantastic. It is expected that emissions will fall by an unprecedented 8% this year. Daily emissions in April fell by17% (Guardian May 20th). This does not mean we have solved the problem of climate change, but we have given the planet a chance to breathe for a moment.

Whether we take this crisis as a divine signal that we need to change our ways or just use our gifts of common sense, there is one clear lesson to be received and carefully digested: nature is far stronger than human organisation. China and Italy were overwhelmed before they knew it. The U.K. and North America are still reeling and who knows what will happen in India and Sub-Saharan Africa? Nature can knock us down with the flat of its hand without warning. We stagger to our feet and wonder what happened.

As noted above, this is not the first serious epidemic in less than twenty years. It is just the first to become a true pandemic. Wildfires have ripped through California, the Amazon and Australia. Storm systems are on the increase and huge swarms of locusts are threatening East-Africa with famine. Do we need reminding that the human race is under threat?

Maybe we do. Maybe we needed to be forced to take a pause and wake up. Climate change is accelerating. Sea level rise is no-longer a computer model. Pacific Islands are disappearing and agricultural land in low lying coastal areas is being lost to salt water. Glaciers are shrinking at a faster and faster rate. We must not ignore the ways in which our natural environment is being transformed around us. Covid-19 shows exactly what happens when we ignore nature: we are overwhelmed.

Our new world must take climate change into account. Mr Donald Trump says he will not forget the oil industry. In fact, we need to do exactly that: consign it to history. Of course, we cannot leave oil overnight. We need to transition carefully, but this is our opportunity. Crises jolt people into action. They become creative. Possibilities open up. They help us to say goodbye to the old and embrace the new.

As we reconstruct economic life, let us employ strategic thinking to incorporate new and creative technologies and approaches to living into a sustainable future. It used to be said that sustainable energy is too expensive and not reliable. The first is patently no-longer true: year on year a greater proportion of the world's energy comes from renewables. At early stages of technology transition, it is often only the early adopters who think change is possible. People thought the horse would never be replaced by the train and the motorcar. Typewriters were indispensable office equipment and every family would always need a landline. Yet, the world changed.

If investment is created by the pooling of international financial resources, it will be a perfect time to invest in renewable energy and radically reduce our reliance on fossil fuels. In this energy hungry world, clean, sustainable energy production is a source of confidence for the investing world. Strategic, creative, research, development and production can build a new future. It is at this time of challenge when we have seen the failure of our old system that we can jump on board a new environmentally sustainable engine of growth.

Chapter 10
Two Stories ... Two Scenarios.

First Story

Daniel Raj Patel felt totally exhausted as he drifted through the nearly abandoned Ahmedabad International Airport. Black crows nested freely on the steel girders around the smeared windows.

The few passengers on his flight had been carefully spaced out around the plane. All had been tested before boarding and were presumed free of the virus, so there was no insistence on the use of face masks. Daniel was tested again at immigration and had put on his facemask by the time he exited into the arrival's hall. Nobody was there to greet him, and the shops were all closed. An official waved him quickly through and out into the hot Indian sun. He was home, or nearly. A few taxis were waiting at some distance from each other. He took the first one on the rank and was whisked through near empty streets to Maninagar East. He had phoned his wife on landing and found her with his daughters waiting behind the gate to his compound.

Inside, his favourite armchair enfolded him in its loving embrace as his family fussed around … chai … idli … bhujia … spicy chicken wings … all his favourites. The girls sat around him, trying to look engrossed in their electronic devices, but he knew they wanted to know what had happened at the conference. Daniel opened his eyes and smiled. Their mother refilled his chai and asked them to let him rest.

"No, no, my dear. It is rest enough that I am home." He touched her hand and she pecked his cheek before disappearing back into the kitchen.

"Well, my dears, we still have a long way to go, but I think we have made some progress on the way…"

The International Health and Economic Renewal Conference in August 2020 nearly failed to take place. The timetable was extremely tight, and the Americans had insisted that it should be under the auspices of the G20 not the United Nations, which upset nearly everyone. At first a virtual conference was proposed, but it was soon clear that this would allow too much room for public posturing in front of the world's media.

With accommodation for up to 23,000 participants, Davos was chosen as the venue and it was agreed that there should be a media lockdown for the whole 14-day conference. Only at the end of the last day were selected news organisation representatives flown in. The media had exploded with indignation, but the unprecedented situation and demands of political leaders forced them to accept it. At the last minute the American and Chinese dispute over the causes and early handling of the Covid-19 emergency nearly derailed everything, but after a mysterious eleventh hour phone call between Presidents Trump and Putin, the Americans seemed to forget the issue and final planning for joint international security arrangements went ahead. On 14th August the conference opened.

Daniel sketched out his role in helping to co-ordinate the re-writing of pandemic management protocols in the light of Covid-19 experience and outlines for public healthcare systems focused on epidemiological threats. International experts had had little trouble agreeing on what to do. Yet, despite this success, the first few days saw political chaos. Hollow speeches of good intent echoed around the conference chambers as proposals for concrete action were repeatedly rejected behind closed doors. After three days, bridges between entrenched positions were getting harder to build. Daniel had begun to despair. Small groups of delegates sat drinking late into the night, fearful of what the next day might bring.

As part of the conference, organisers had reluctantly allowed one of the 58 conference hotels to be used as the venue for a parallel meeting of world spiritual representatives. The major leaders of the world's faiths were present, as well as representatives of smaller faith communities. Two of them, representing different spiritual traditions had each somehow managed to bring one of their children. These insignificant seven-year olds, Sunita and Philip, sat quietly together during meetings, each with a drawing book and pencils. Nobody paid them much attention, except occasionally to drop by and praise their work, which always in some way centred on the drawing of a single star. Discussions about the teachings of Jesus, Mohammed, Buddha and many more failed completely to disturb their concentration. Only at the prayer times, set at five intervals during the day, did they put their colours to one side.

On the fourth evening a plenary session had been scheduled in the main auditorium to review progress. Health experts and economists spoke with enthusiasm of their plans. Then it was time for the political leaders. Donald Trump rose and strode to the platform; his demeanour did not bode well. He slammed his papers down on the lectern and eyed the audience malignantly.

"The United States of America came here to lead our dear world out of this crisis. We are the economic and military power that can do this, if you will let us. We are the best and we offer you the best. But in the last 4 days we have found that the liberals and socialists and communists of this world have refused to submit to us…"

A murmur of discontent began to gather.

"We have a road-map to rebuild our world and return us to prosperity. Tonight, I give you your last chance to join us. Unless I hear by nine o'clock tomorrow morning…"

Delegates began to fold their papers, gather their electronic devices and move towards the exits.

Trump stopped in mid-sentence as a beam of light struck the podium through the now dark windows. From the back of the hall came two small children holding brightly coloured pictures of stars above their heads. A hush descended as people were pulled back to their seats.

Trump began again. "There is no option for the world, but to …."

A gentle communal "shush" quietly filled the auditorium. The children reached the platform and sat on the steps holding the pictures above their heads, their backs bathed in light.

Trump's shadow loomed monstrously over his audience as the auditorium windows overlooking the Davos valley filled with light. Turning, and shielding his eyes, he saw its source falling precipitously before him. The comet's tail bathed the whole valley in gold. For the first time in his life Daniel realised what it meant for silence to be golden.

It held them all. Whether it was for hours, minutes or seconds no-one knew, but a presence had spoken. Then it was gone. The delegates exhaled a communal sigh of relief, wonder and awe. No-one spoke. Donald Trump shook his head and almost crept out of a side door. People slowly began to move. Attempts to speak were met with quiet rebuttals, as everyone left, except for the two children. They looked at each other, lowered their pictures, massaged their tired arms, giggled and walked out.

Next morning the five permanent members of the UN Security Council met over breakfast. By the end of the day an outline health and economic security package had been agreed by the whole council. The next two days saw the details being hammered out by the rest of the conference delegates.

By the end of the first week a World Health Executive had been created with power to oversee the prevention and treatment of epidemiological diseases worldwide. In addition, the world's gold reserves had been pooled as the basis for a global wealth fund which could back the creation of Covid-19 recovery bonds overseen by a new International Recovery Bank…...

"So Dad, the conference was a success. You've saved the world!" Jashmitha responded excitedly.

Daniel smiled as he eased himself up and made for his bedroom. "Yes, we've made a start. But only time will tell…..and if anyone phones tell them I don't exist."

<u>Five years Later</u>

Jashmitha slipped her key into the lock, almost fell over the threshold of her apartment and came to rest on the living room sofa on top of a multicoloured sari.

"Hey Jash, that's my wedding sari. I've just ironed it." Samira pushed her sister off the heavy silk fabric and marched off to her room.

Jashmitha allowed her body to slide to the floor. She felt like she might never move again.

"Samira, don't treat your sister like that. She's just finished a week of twelve-hour shifts, so she can be at your wedding." Mrs Patel appeared with a chai and helped her daughter back onto the sofa. "Come and say sorry."

A head appeared briefly round the door frame, "sorry, sis," and disappeared.

By the end of the following day Samira would be the happy bride of Sanjay Gupta, proprietor of a small start-up windfarm enterprise in Rajasthan. Like many others he had been given venture capital by the *Jindal Foundation* and now employed over a hundred former day labourers in tending his turbines and running small enterprises which used the cheap power his company produced.

Jashmitha had followed her father into epidemiology, working at an infectious disease unit. Puji slid onto the sofa and stroked her sister's arm. How was it? You look a wreck.

"I think we're winning. There are only two cases of Ebola 2 and five of swine flu. We think we've found and isolated all contacts and there haven't been any new cases of either identified for ten days."

"You were lucky to find the ones you got."

"Not really, our airport testing is so good. Nobody gets through. Dad saw to that," replied Jashmitha. Their mother crouched on the floor beside them, a tear rolling down her cheek.

"Your father was a great man, even if he did let them kill him with hard work. Don't let them do the same to you, girl, you've got a lot of life to live yet."

"I know. I know. I'll be careful. I hope they realise how much India has to thank Dad for. Our testing and tracing is second to none and our vaccine development is a world beater. We've got contracts with 66 countries and now we're helping some of them to set up their own facilities. The UK is learning from us."

Samira strode in with the TV remote and CNN burst into life. Boris Johnson had secured a second term, by splitting his party and embracing liberal socialism. A funeral cortege was snaking through the streets of Washington. Donald Trump had won his second term, but had been a changed man. Gone were the bluster and defiance. As his base faded away, the country swung behind an enfeebled old patriot, with a far-away look in his eye, who reminded people of the American dream. He was dead soon after inauguration and his vice-president was found to have cancer and now was on his last journey. A new leader of the House of Representatives was now president and the red necks were boiling for a fight.

The business reporter announced encouraging second quarter profits in both North America and Europe. Stocks in renewables were riding high as oil companies began to bite the bullet and diversify.

Life was a struggle, but ok. The girls muted the T.V. and turned their minds to the wedding.

Second Story

Ghita sat in her kitchen on a hard, wooden stool, nursing a cup of chai. A pan was simmering gently on the stove, so she could serve her husband as soon as he came in. He should have finished his hospital shift at 11.00pm and it was after 1.00am. He was long over-due, and Ahmedabad was becoming increasingly unsafe at night. Ghita had sent her three daughters, Jashmitha, Samira and Puji to bed. They had to be up early for school and college, but she knew they wouldn't be sleeping. Jashmitha slipped quietly into the kitchen, helped herself to some chai and held her mother's hand across the kitchen table. Dad had phoned about midnight to say he had been kept late, but was on his way. The doctors were overwhelmed with more Covid-19 cases.

They were shocked to their feet by heavy thumping on the apartment door and ran to open it. Two police officers stood there holding their father, whose face was covered in blood. They lurched forward, dragging their charge. "Where?" gasped the first man in a blood-stained uniform. "In here, on the sofa, gasped Jashmitha," as her mother grabbed some towels and filled a bowl with water. "Lock your door," shouted the second officer as he left, "the mob saw us coming in here. They're blaming the doctors."

Ghita knelt and bathed her husband's head. The blood had clotted. Jashmitha found some antiseptic in the bathroom and applied it to the wounds. She was in her second year of medicine and was pretty sure the injuries were only superficial. Daniel Raj Patel opened his eyes slightly, raised his hand and felt for his wife's face.

Cleaned up and bandaged, Daniel sat over his breakfast cleaning his plate with roti until it shone. The view from the window looked quite normal, except for a few plumes of smoke rising in the distance and some burned out cars in the street.

"I hate to say it, but we'll have to leave. The government is losing control. The people have lost faith in us. People say they're starving in the villages and are on their way back to the cities to take what they can. I don't blame them either."

"What about Sanjay?" Cried Samira.

"He's only the boy next door. It's not like you're promised to each other," said her mother quietly.

"We love each other. We always have."

Daniel gave his wife a stern look. "I'll speak to Sanjay's father today. I know he's worried, but I can't promise anything."

Samira fingered her phone. "I could speak to them now."

"Let me handle it. He's their only son. We could all go together. It might be better that way."

Daniel rose to go, but his wife took his hand firmly and pulled him back. "Where can we go, dear? We don't know anyone in Delhi."

"I know some of Modi's men. They might help, but I think we need to leave India until things settle down."

"Leave India, Papa. You can't be serious. It's our life. Everything. And where will we go?" Jashmitha couldn't believe what she was hearing.

Daniel replied, "this is all happening so suddenly. I would never have believed I could say such things, but after last night, I think it's a matter of life or death. We could go to China. My knowledge might be worth something there, or Africa. With their experience with Ebola, they're doing better than many people expected. I think we'd be safe there and they certainly need doctors."

He left the family in stunned silence to go and talk to their next-door neighbour. Four days later they were in two Toyota Hilux vans, booked on a flight to Nairobi with as much luggage as the plane allowed. Samira and Sanjay sat like star-crossed lovers; fingers tightly entwined.

Getting plane tickets and entry visas had not been easy, but a doctor and a health science engineer and his university professor wife were valued commodities. Daniel was well enough known on the international epidemiology circuit. He had picked up a newspaper in the airport terminal and began to read it as they settled into their flight. Ghita and Sanjay's mother were deep in conversation, even through their face masks.

The news was not good. The Indian treasury had announced that it had no more money to provide food for the poor. Its borrowing would have to be curtailed in order to support the Rupee. "Fiscal common sense must prevail until the crisis is over." The IMF and World Bank were not in a position to help "as the present situation does not meet their lending criteria."

The plane lurched to one side and the cabin service director announced that due to turbulence normal cabin service would be suspended. It seemed to be a metaphor for real life.

He turned to international news. The death toll in Canada was under control, but in the United States it was still climbing steeply. Policy had now been placed entirely in the hands of state governors. Some states were doing well, while in others the virus was still rampant. No-one seemed willing to learn from anyone else, while the rhetoric at the international level was out of control.

Buried on the newspaper's penultimate page was an offer by Switzerland to host an international health and reconstruction conference at Davos. President Trump had responded that there was no point until China agreed that they were responsible for the pandemic and paid compensation. China would attend, but needed firm financial commitments from the U.S.A. before it agreed. Russia made no public comment. Daniel was pleased to see that deaths were down in Europe, but with so little international cooperation he feared for the future. It would be better to hide in Africa for a while, and leave the rest of the world alone. What a terrible way of thinking.

<u>Five Years Later</u>

"To our daughter, Jashmitha Patel, congratulations on your qualification as a medical doctor. May God bless you and give you a wonderful career." The little group of smartly dressed Indians, plus two young African men, raised their glasses of red wine and Jashmitha pretended to be a shy little girl. No-one believed her act for one moment.

Settling into Nairobi had not been easy, but five years on, the two families were well established and seemed to have been accepted in Africa. Their secret was that they had really learned to value their new continent. It had saved their lives and they were thankful. At the same time, they were devastated by nearly every piece of news from India. The second half of 2020 had seen widespread destruction and looting in every town and city. Only Delhi had been saved ……by the army. Elsewhere there were not enough troops and the death toll amongst the police was horrific. As 2021 progressed and things got no better, India was persuaded to accept military help from China to re-establish law and order. Agriculture and Industry needed huge cash support, which China was willing to give, at a price.

Further afield, life was finding a new normal. The European Union had been through a shaky time. Some sudden exits had shaken the rest of the club into renewed cooperation and with new Eurobonds, recovery was creaking along. Britain was struggling on alone and had had four governments in as many years, but a new Health and Welfare Council had kept the country free of both Ebola 2 and Swine Flu, which could not be said for North America.

Daniel paid the bill and led the group out into Nairobi's traffic. An hour later they were back at their apartment building. Samira and Sanjay immediately disappeared. A month into marriage, they were aching for intimacy. The remainder of the two families squeezed themselves into an elevator which clanked its way up to their tenth-floor apartments.

Once home, the girls left their parents facing each other by the living room window. Ghita held her husband's upper arms and kissed his lips lightly.

"We aren't doing so badly, considering everything, are we? It was a lovely occasion. Thank you. Sam and Sanjay are so in love. It's beautiful."

"Yes, my dear, do you remember when we were like that? My mother told me to be careful because you'd love me to death." replied Daniel. "I think Paul and Jashmitha are not far off. He's a good boy. So respectful."

"Mm, he knows what he wants, but does he know what he's getting? Sash is so independent. She'll want the driving seat." Ghita smiled, pecked Daniel's cheek and went to make chai.

Daniel found his newspaper and put his feet up on the sofa. At least all seemed well with his world.

"Dad, Dad, Paul just texted me" Jashmitha hurtled into the room, pushed her father's feet off the sofa and pressed herself into his side. "It's all over the news. The Americans are blaming the Chinese for swine flu and Ebola 2 and are threatening to withdraw from the United Nations."

Daniel grabbed the TV remote and found CNN.

"…moving so fast that we can hardly keep up. A Pentagon spokesman says they have reliable information of China's secret biological weapons programme and have instructed the United States Seventh Fleet to deploy in the South China Sea."

Daniel switched it off.

"Dad!"

He hugged his daughter. "I can't watch it. It takes me back to the fear I felt that night back home when I thought I'd never see you all again."

Ghita silently placed two cups of chai on the table, settled into the armchair at his side, and took his hand. "We'll make it through, dear. The world will live again."

Part Three
Building Change

Chapter 11
Manifesto for Sustainable Change

As I have looked at this crisis, I have sought to identify policies that will help us to build a sustainable future. As I close, I want to bring these together in summary. These are broad brush recommendations. Application requires careful tailoring to specific situations, but they form a firm foundation for future prosperity.

1. Strategic focus that people are the core of global life.
   - o Economic life that protects and enhances the lives of ordinary people and communities.

- o People to be valued as creative resources, not dispensable economic fodder.

2. Governments must engage in strategic economic planning, in order to safeguard the lives of the people.
   - o Protection of vital industries, national skill reservoirs and supply chains.
   - o Protection of food supply chains and crop diversity.
   - o Public investment in infrastructure to underwrite economic renewal.
   - o Investment in renewable energy, recycling and new sustainable industries committed to environmental renewal.

3. Countries must engage in international cooperation for the sake of world economic renewal.
   - o Pooling of national financial resources to underwrite a system of 10- year Covid-19 bonds to boost global public spending on industrial renewal.

4. Creative entrepreneurial energy needs to be released in individuals and communities, stimulated and supported by public and private capital.
   - o Local and regional regeneration networks to stimulate creative entrepreneurship.

5. Parallel national health systems need to be created
   in order to protect general health needs from being
   undermined when epidemiological crises occur.
   - o Creation of an epidemiology focused public
     health system resourced and prepared to
     meet the needs of future epidemics and
     health crises.
   - o A general healthcare system separate from
     epidemiological provision.
6. An independent international health agency, created
   by an international treaty, should oversee global
   epidemiological research and health provision.
   - o Proactive investigation of viruses and other
     pathogens which may have jumped or be
     likely to jump the species barrier (Zoonotic
     infections).
   - o Active, on-going development of vaccines.
   - o Development of agreed protocols for dealing
     with possible epidemics structured around
     testing, tracing and isolating cases.
7. Return to normal socialisation and economic life
   needs to be facilitated by development of testing
   and tracing technology as an urgent priority.
   - o Mass, easily available Covid-19 testing to
     facilitate the re-establishment of social and
     economic life.

The Age of Struggle

Periods of history have often been characterised by defining phenomena. The 18th Century *Age of Reason* dispensed with many of the superstitions and mystical apprehensions of the medieval mind. The 19th Century saw the *Age of Empire* as European hegemony dominated the globe. The 20th Century has been described as the *Age of Social Transformation.* What will our age be known for?

I dare to suggest that we have entered *The Age of Struggle.* This is not to say that history or indeed every human life is not full of struggles. Hegel saw history as a dialectical struggle of thesis and antithesis spawning new realities and in turn new antitheses.

Yet with postmodernism we seem to have entered a new age of struggle. Gone are the old overarching certainties of modernism, in the guise of socialism or capitalism. As climate change takes hold and in the face of Covid-19 and other health crises, we are struggling to find a road map into a sustainable future. In the midst of uncertainty, politics is often rudderless. People swing this way and that, grasping at the latest messiah. One seems to hark back to a mythical past of old certainties, while another presents impossible dreams of prosperity. When the messiah is found to have feet of clay, electorates swing away to find someone else or vent their discontent in other ways. We are struggling to find our way into the future. There is not even agreement about what it should look like.

The muddle of national and international politics is so profound that the leadership that the world needs today is not being allowed to emerge. Emmanuel Macron arose as the face of a new future in France and Europe, only to lose his popularity almost as soon as he began to wield power and has been almost overwhelmed by the Yellow Vest Movement. Two men in their 70s are vying for supreme power in the United States. Russia and China both have increasingly authoritarian one-party rule by leaders clinging to power. Much of the Middle East has been destroyed by military adventurism and Turkey has its own struggle between authoritarian fundamentalism and secular democracy. In many parts of the world illiberal populism has created toxic narratives inflamed by amoral use of social media for political advantage. The voice of considered reason based on science and tested empirical observation is often shouted down by midnight tweets and ill-considered soundbites.

This is also the *Age of Struggle* in another very important sense. It is the age in which those who reject illiberal populist xenophobia must embrace world-wide community of purpose and make their voices heard. If this *Manifesto for a Sustainable Future* is put into effect, it will be because the people of the world grasp hold of it and make it happen. The International Community needs to come together and lobby for people centred health systems, people centred economic renewal and people centred strategic vision. We will have to struggle for the creation of a multinational health infrastructure to keep the world safe from future pandemics. We must engage locally, nationally and internationally to create the strategic economic paradigms and structures which will form a basis for economic renewal. Only then will we bring public and private capital together in a coalition of creative enterprise.

So, after Covid-19…What? Crises can lead to pessimistic retreat into our own pain, as we cast around for those to blame from behind xenophobic walls, or they can promote creative engagement and problem solving in order to challenge the crisis and build the future. The struggle is on between these two paradigms. During lockdown, so many people have reached out to each other in caring creativity that it is clear humanity ultimately has the strength to win through. Yet, we need actively and intentionally to embrace the values of people centred, strategic multinationalism, if we are going to build a sustainable global future.

Sources

- American Society for Micro-biology
  - https://www.asm.org/
- Coalition for Epidemic Preparedness Innovations (CEPI)
  - https://cepi.net/
- Centers for Disease Control and Prevention (U.S.)
  - https://www.cdc.gov/
- Guardian News and Media
  - https://www.theguardian.com
- International Monetary Fund
  - www.imf.org
- National Centre for Biotechnology Information
  - https://www.ncbi.nlm.nih.gov/
- Nature Medicine
  - https://www.nature.com/nm/
- The Journal of Medical Virology
  - https://onlinelibrary.wiley.com/journal/10969071

- The Lancet
    - https://www.thelancet.com/
- Wikipedia
    - https://en.wikipedia.org
- World Health Organisation
    - https://www.who.int/
- Worldometer
    - https://www.worldometers.info/coronavirus/
- Vox.com
    - https://www.vox.com/